The Complete Diabetes Code

Everything You Need to Know About Diabetes

By 

Dr. David R. Wheat

TABLE OF CONTENTS

Introduction

If it hasn't already, the rate at which diabetes is being passed around suggests that it may soon become an epidemic. The number of people being diagnosed with diabetes is increasing at an alarming rate.

The most significant contributors to diabetes in younger and middle-aged people are a sedentary lifestyle and bad eating habits, which are two of the many underlying causes of the disease.

In many situations, it gives birth to diabesity, which is a combination of diabetes and obesity that has a substantial impact on life and longevity.

Diabetes, with all of its associated issues, can impair one's quality of life and lead to an increase in stress due to the have to continually check one's blood sugar levels, eat a limited diet, and take medication every day.

Modifications to one's way of life and one's diet, in particular, have the potential to cut one's risk of developing diabetes by a sizeable percentage.

People frequently think of infectious diseases like SARS, HIV, or the flu when they hear the word "epidemic."

On the other hand, the incidence of type 2 diabetes has recently reached epidemic levels.

The Complete Diabetes Code

Diabetes is the sixth greatest cause of death in the United States, and it is responsible for more than 130 billion dollars worth of costs associated with health care.
The number of newly identified instances of the disease continues to climb.
It is anticipated that one out of every three children who entered the world in the year 2000 may get diabetes at some point during their lives.
Diabetes is expected to become one of the most frequent diseases in the world during the next couple of decades, affecting at least half a billion people. This prediction was made by researchers.

The increasing rate of obesity in the general population is the primary contributor to the alarmingly high diabetes diagnosis rate.
In today's culture, it might be challenging to keep up a healthy weight and lifestyle. We also have rather sedentary lifestyles, which contribute to our weight gain.
This stands in stark contrast to life only a couple of hundred years ago, when people were much more physically active, and there was a scarcity of food supplies. As a direct consequence of this, many of us are currently carrying excess weight.

The Complete Diabetes Code

Bringing attention to the devastating effects of diabetes may also encourage society as a whole to take action to halt the spread of the disease and improve the lives of those who are afflicted with it on a day-to-day basis. The collaborative efforts of multiple groups—including the government, industry, medical professionals, nutritionists, and people whose lives have been affected by diabetes—will contribute to the reduction of the diabetes pandemic, the limitation of its effects, and the guarantee of excellent health for a variety of populations.
The Complete Diabetes Code takes into account any and all non-pharmaceutical and inexpensive methods of combating the diabetes epidemic.

Get rid of this silent killer disease by getting your copy of this book right now!

Chapter 1
Diabetes

Diabetes is a long-term condition (a chronic disease) that manifests itself either when the pancreas loses its ability to create insulin or when the body is unable to make effective use of the insulin that it does produce.

Insulin is a hormone that is produced by the pancreas. It performs the function of a key by allowing glucose, which comes from the food that we eat, to move from the bloodstream into the cells of the body, where it may be converted into energy. In the body, glucose is produced through the digestion of any food that contains carbohydrates. Insulin facilitates the entry of glucose into the cells.

If you have diabetes, your body either is unable to produce enough insulin or is unable to utilize it as effectively as it can. When there is not enough insulin or when cells cease responding to insulin, an excessive amount of blood sugar remains in the bloodstream. This condition is known as diabetes. This can, over time, lead to major health issues such as coronary heart disease, eyesight loss, and kidney disease.

The Complete Diabetes Code

The primary culprit behind each form of diabetes is something different. However, if you have diabetes of any kind, it can cause you to have an excessive amount of sugar in your blood. The presence of unhealthy levels of sugar in the blood might result in major health issues. Both type 1 and type 2 diabetes are examples of diseases that can lead to chronic diabetes.

Prediabetes and diabetes that develops during pregnancy are two forms of diabetes that have the potential to be reversed. When a person's blood sugar levels are higher than what is considered normal, they are said to have prediabetes. However, the levels of glucose in the blood are not high enough to diagnose the condition as diabetes. And if actions aren't taken to prevent diabetes, prediabetes can develop into full-blown diabetes. Diabetes mellitus during pregnancy is referred to as gestational diabetes. However, it is possible that it may disappear after the baby is born.

Types of Diabetes

Type 1 Diabetes

It is believed that an autoimmune reaction is what causes this particular form of diabetes (the body attacks itself by mistake). Because of this reaction, your body will no longer produce insulin. Type 1 diabetes affects around 5–10% of those who are diagnosed with diabetes. Diabetes type 1 frequently manifests itself with rapid onset of symptoms. In most cases, the diagnosis is made in younger people, including children, adolescents, and young adults. If you have type 1 diabetes, you will need to inject insulin into your body on a daily basis in order to stay alive. At the moment, there is no one who knows how to stop type 1 diabetes.

Type 2 Diabetes

This type of diabetes affects adults more frequently than children and accounts for around 90 per cent of all occurrences of diabetes. In people who have type 2 diabetes, their bodies are unable to make effective use of the insulin that they produce. A healthy lifestyle, consisting of higher levels of physical activity and a nutritious diet, is the primary component in the treatment of type 2 diabetes.

However, over time, the majority of people who have type 2 diabetes will require the use of oral medications and/or insulin in order to maintain control of their blood glucose levels.

Gestational Diabetes

Gestational diabetes is a type of diabetes that only affects pregnant women who have never before struggled with diabetes. If you have gestational diabetes, there is a greater possibility that your baby will have health complications. Diabetes that develops during pregnancy may typically disappear after the delivery of the baby. On the other hand, it raises the probability that you may develop type 2 diabetes in later life. If your newborn is overweight, they have a greater chance of becoming obese as children or teenagers and developing type 2 diabetes later in life.

Symptoms

The severity of diabetes symptoms is directly related to how high a person's blood sugar level is. It's possible that some people, particularly those who have prediabetes or type 2 diabetes, won't show any symptoms at all. Diabetes type 1 is characterized by symptoms that develop more rapidly and are more severe.

The Complete Diabetes Code

The following are some of the symptoms that are associated with type 1 diabetes and type 2 diabetes:
1. Experiencing a greater thirst than normal.
2. Having to urinate frequently.
3. Shedding pounds without making any effort to do so.
4. The demonstration of ketone bodies in the urine. Ketones are a result of the breakdown of muscle and fat that occurs when there is not enough accessible insulin. This process takes place when there is a lack of glucose in the blood.
5. Experiencing lethargy and general weakness.
6. Having irritating feelings or experiencing other shifts in mood.
7. Experiencing vision that is hazy.
8. Suffering from sores that heal quite slowly.
9. Suffering from several infections, including those of the gums, skin, and vaginal cavity.
Diabetes type 1 can develop at any point in a person's life. On the other hand, it frequently begins in childhood or adolescence. At any age, a person is at risk for developing type 2 diabetes, which is the more frequent form. People over the age of 40 have a greater risk of developing type 2 diabetes.

Causes

It is necessary to have an understanding of how the body regularly makes use of glucose in order to comprehend diabetes.

How insulin works:

Insulin is a hormone that is produced by a gland that is located below and behind the stomach (pancreas). Insulin enters the bloodstream as a product of the pancreas' secretion.

Sugar is able to enter the cells because insulin is circulating throughout the body.

Insulin has the effect of reducing the quantity of sugar that is present in the bloodstream.

When there is a decrease in the amount of sugar in the blood, the pancreas responds by producing less insulin.

The role of glucose:

The cells that comprise muscles and other tissues receive their supply of energy from glucose, which is a type of sugar. Food and the liver are the two primary places where glucose can be found. The digestion of sugar results in its entry into the bloodstream, where insulin facilitates its transport to the cells. The glucose is stored in the liver, which also produces it.

The Complete Diabetes Code

After blood glucose levels are low, such as they are when a person has gone several hours without eating, the liver converts glycogen stores into glucose by breaking them down. Your glucose level will remain within the normal range as a result of this.

It is currently uncertain what exactly causes the majority of kinds of diabetes. Sugar accumulates in the bloodstream regardless of the situation.

This is due to an inadequate amount of insulin being produced by the pancreas. Both type 1 and type 2 diabetes may have their origins in a complex web of hereditary and environmental risk factors. It is not quite obvious what those potential factors are.

Diabetes and depression:

Managing both diabetes and depression at the same time can be challenging.

What exactly is the relationship between diabetes and mental illness?

If you have diabetes, either type 1 or type 2, you have a greater chance of acquiring depression. This is true regardless of the type of diabetes you have. In addition, having a history of depression has been linked to an increased risk of acquiring type 2 diabetes.

The good news is that treatment for depression and diabetes can be combined in some patients. And being able to successfully manage one can help with managing the other.

How they're related

Managing diabetes can be stressful and lead to symptoms of depression, despite the fact that the association between depression and diabetes is not well understood. Diabetes can produce difficulties and health problems, both of which have the potential to make depressive symptoms more severe.

Depression can cause a person to make poor choices in their life. Some examples of these are improper eating, decreased physical activity, smoking, and weight gain. Each and every one of these is a diabetes risk factor.

Depression can make it difficult to carry out daily activities, maintain relationships, and think coherently. Because of this, maintaining effective control of diabetes can be challenging.

Taking care of both of these situations simultaneously: Diabetes self-management programs. Diabetes programs that place emphasis on behavior can assist individuals in taking control of their metabolism, enhancing their levels of physical fitness, and managing risk factors for heart disease and weight reduction. Your overall sense of well-being and quality of life may both increase as a result of participating in these activities.

Psychotherapy: People who take part in psychotherapy, particularly cognitive behavioral therapy, have a greater chance of seeing a reduction in their symptoms of depression. They may find that this makes it easier for them to control their diabetes.

Adjustments to diet, exercise, and medication: Both diabetes and depression are treatable diseases that can benefit from lifestyle adjustments and different medications. A variety of therapeutic approaches, in addition to consistent physical activity, are available as choices.

Both depression and diabetes can benefit from collaborative care, which refers to treatment that is overseen by a group of healthcare professionals and that ramps up the amount of therapy when necessary.

It's possible that certain healthcare systems won't provide this kind of treatment to their patients.

If you have diabetes, you should be on the lookout for signs of sadness. These can include a loss of interest in activities that were formerly enjoyable, feelings of despair or hopelessness, and inexplicable physical problems like headaches or back discomfort.

Seek immediate assistance if you are concerned that you may be suffering from depression. Your primary care physician or diabetes educator should be able to assist you in locating a mental health professional.

Risk Factor: Different types of diabetes have different risk factors associated with them. The patient's family history may be a factor in all of the categories. The risk of developing type 1 diabetes can be increased by both environmental and geographical variables.

It is not uncommon for persons with type 1 diabetes to have family members tested to see whether or not they have diabetic immune system cells (autoantibodies). When you have these autoantibodies, your risk of getting type 1 diabetes is significantly elevated. Although some people with these autoantibodies go on to acquire diabetes, others do not.

There is some evidence that a person's race or ethnicity can increase their likelihood of getting type 2 diabetes. Certain persons, such as those who are Black, Hispanic, American Indian, or Asian American, are at a higher risk, although the reasons for this are not completely understood.

People who are overweight or obese have a significantly increased risk of developing prediabetes, type 2 diabetes, and gestational diabetes.

Long-term complications of diabetes develop gradually: Diabetes causes progressive progression of long-term consequences, including the following: Complications of diabetes become more likely the longer a person has the disease and the less effective their blood sugar is managed. In the long run, problems from diabetes could render a person unable to work or even put their life in jeopardy. Prediabetes is a condition that can develop into type 2 diabetes. Possible complications include: The disease of the heart and blood vessels (also known as cardiovascular disease). Diabetes significantly raises the risk of a variety of heart-related complications. These conditions can include coronary artery disease with chest pain (also known as angina), a heart attack, a stroke, and constriction of the arteries (atherosclerosis).

Diabetes puts a person at an increased risk of developing cardiovascular disease and stroke.

Nerve damage (neuropathy): Can occur when an excessive amount of sugar is consumed. This can destroy the walls of the capillaries, which are the very small blood vessels that supply nutrition to the nerves, particularly in the legs. This might result in sensations such as tingling, numbness, burning, or pain that typically start at the extremities, such as the tips of the toes or fingers, and progressively move upward.

When the nerves that are responsible for digestion are damaged, it can lead to difficulties with nausea, vomiting, diarrhea, or constipation. It is possible that men who experience this will develop erectile dysfunction.

Kidney damage (nephropathy): Kidneys contain millions of microscopic blood artery clusters called glomeruli, which filter waste out of the blood. This fragile filtering system is susceptible to harm from diabetes.

Eye damage (retinopathy): Is a term that refers to damage that diabetes can cause to the retina's blood vessels (diabetic retinopathy). This could result in permanent vision loss.

Foot damage: the risk of various foot issues is increased when there is nerve damage in the feet or when there is the insufficient blood supply to the feet.

Skin and mouth conditions: Diabetes might make you more susceptible to skin problems, including bacterial and fungal infections, as well as oral diseases. Diabetes can also make you more likely to experience dry mouth.

Hearing impairment: Diabetes patients are more likely to experience hearing issues than the general population.

Alzheimer's disease: Diabetes type 2 has been linked to an increased chance of developing dementia, including Alzheimer's disease.

Depression: Depression is a typical complication for those who suffer from diabetes, both type 1 and type 2.

Complications of gestational diabetes: The vast majority of healthy babies are delivered by mothers who have gestational diabetes. However, if your blood sugar levels are not addressed or controlled, it could lead to complications for both you and your baby. Gestational diabetes can lead to a number of complications for your unborn child, including the following:

Out-of-control growth. Additional glucose is able to pass through the placenta. The pancreas of the newborn will produce additional insulin when there is an excess of glucose. Your child's size may become unhealthily enormous as a result of this. It may result in the necessity for a difficult delivery or even a cesarean section in some cases.

Low blood sugar. Babies born to moms who have gestational diabetes may experience low blood sugar (hypoglycemia) in the first few hours or days of their lives. This is because their body produces a significant amount of insulin already.

Diabetes type 2 developed in later life. Children born to moms who suffer from gestational diabetes have an increased likelihood of becoming obese and getting type 2 diabetes in later life.

Death. If gestational diabetes is not treated, it might result in the death of the baby either before or shortly after it is born.

Gestational diabetes. Gestational diabetes can potentially lead to complications for the mother, including the following complications:

Amputation and diabetes. High blood pressure, an abnormally high level of protein in the urine, and swelling in the lower extremities are some of the symptoms of this illness.

Diabetes mellitus in pregnancy. If you previously experienced gestational diabetes during pregnancy, you have an increased risk of developing it again during a subsequent pregnancy.

Diabetes and amputations go hand in hand.

diabetes-related complications affecting the bones and joints

Display more information that is relevant.

Prevention

Diabetes type 1 cannot be avoided in any way. However, the same changes in lifestyle that can help cure prediabetes, type 2 diabetes, and gestational diabetes can also help avoid these conditions:

Consume only nutritious foods. Pick foods that are lower in fat and calories and higher in fiber rather than vice versa. Put your emphasis on fruits, vegetables, and grains that are whole. Consume a wide variety of foods to prevent feelings of monotony.

Increase the amount of physical exercise you do.

Make it a goal to participate in some form of aerobic activity for around half an hour on most days of the week. Or, set a weekly goal of engaging in aerobic activity for at least one hundred fifty minutes at a moderate intensity. As an illustration, go for a quick walk every day. If you are unable to commit to a lengthy workout session, you should instead divide it up into several shorter sessions that you perform throughout the day.

Get rid of those extra pounds. If you are overweight, decreasing as little as 7% of your body weight can significantly reduce the likelihood that you will get diabetes. A person who weighs 200 pounds (90.7 kilograms), for instance, may be able to reduce their chance of developing diabetes by dropping 14 pounds (6.4 kilograms).

You should not make an effort to reduce your weight while you are pregnant. Have a conversation with your healthcare practitioner about the appropriate amount of weight gain for you to have during your pregnancy.

Work on making modifications to your food and exercise routines that are meant to be long-term if you want to maintain a healthy weight.

The Complete Diabetes Code

Keep in mind the many advantages of achieving a healthy weight, such as having a healthier heart, greater energy, and a higher sense of self-worth.

There are situations when medicines can be an option. Metformin (Glumetza, Fortamet, and others) and other oral diabetes medications may reduce the likelihood of developing type 2 diabetes. Nevertheless, making healthy lifestyle choices is essential. If you have prediabetes, getting your blood sugar checked at least once a year to ensure that you have not progressed to type 2 diabetes is very important.

Chapter 2
What Happens Inside Your Body When You Eat

Your body will produce an increase in blood glucose that is not good when you consume an excessive amount of calories and fat. If blood glucose is not maintained under control, it can lead to major difficulties, such as hyperglycemia, which, if it is allowed to remain, can lead to long-term complications, such as damage to the nerves, kidneys, and heart. If blood glucose is not kept under control, it can lead to serious problems.

A diet for diabetes is nothing more than consuming the healthiest foods possible in appropriate portions and maintaining a consistent eating schedule.

A healthy eating plan that is naturally abundant in nutrients and low in fat and calories is an example of a diabetes diet. Fruits, vegetables, and grains in their entire form are essential components. In point of fact, a diabetes diet is the most beneficial eating plan for the vast majority of people.

Why should you make an effort to design a plan for healthy eating?

If you have diabetes or prediabetes, your primary care physician will most likely suggest that you consult with a nutritionist so that they can assist you in formulating a healthy eating plan.

The plan assists you in regulating your blood sugar (glucose), helping you maintain a healthy weight, and controlling risk factors for cardiovascular diseases, such as high blood pressure and elevated blood fats.

Your body will produce an increase in blood glucose that is not good when you consume an excessive number of calories and fat. If blood glucose is not maintained under control, it can lead to major difficulties, such as hyperglycemia, which, if it is allowed to remain, can lead to long-term complications, such as damage to the nerves, kidneys, and heart. If blood glucose is not kept under control, it can lead to serious problems.

By paying attention to the foods you eat and choosing nutritious options, you can assist in maintaining a blood glucose level that is within a healthy range.

In most people with type 2 diabetes, losing weight can make it easier to control blood glucose levels and offers a number of other health benefits.

This is in addition to the fact that losing weight can make it simpler to control blood glucose levels. If you want to attain your weight loss goal in a healthy way, following a diabetes diet can give you a well-organized and satisfying path to get there.

What Does a Diabetes Diet Involve?

A diet that targets diabetes emphasizes eating three meals each day at predetermined intervals. This facilitates more effective utilization of the insulin that either your body naturally makes or that you obtain through medication.

A licensed dietician can work with you to develop a diet that takes into account your preferences, as well as your current and future health needs.

You can also have a conversation with him or her about how to improve your eating habits, such as selecting portion sizes that are appropriate for your body size and the amount of activity you engage in.

Recommended Foods:

Utilize these nutrient-dense foods to get the most out of your daily calorie budget. Choose meals that are high in fiber, healthy carbs, seafood, and fats that are considered to be "good."

Healthy carbohydrates

Sugars, which are classified as simple carbohydrates, and starches, which are classified as complex carbs, are both broken down into glucose in the blood after digestion. Put your attention on sources of carbs that are good for you, such as:

Vegetables, Grains that are whole, Legumes, including beans, peas, and other legumes, dairy items, such as milk and cheese that are low in fat.

Steer clear of carbohydrates that aren't as good for you, such as foods or drinks that have extra fat, sugar, or sodium added to them.

Foods that are high in fiber:

All of the portions of plant meals that your body is unable to digest or absorb are included in the definition of dietary fiber. Your body's ability to digest food is tempered by fiber, which also assists in maintaining stable blood sugar levels.

Examples of foods that are high in fiber include:

Vegetables \fruits, Nuts, Legumes, including beans, peas, and other legumes, Grains that are whole

Heart-healthy fish: Fish is good for your heart, so try to eat it at least twice a week.

The consumption of fish high in omega-3 fatty acids, such as salmon, mackerel, tuna, and sardines, may reduce the risk of developing heart disease.

Stay away from fried fish and fish that are known to have high mercury levels, such as king mackerel.

'Good' fats: Consuming more foods that are rich in monounsaturated and polyunsaturated fats will assist in bringing down your overall cholesterol levels. These are the following:

Avocados, Nuts, oils derived from canola, olive, and peanuts. However, moderation is key because every type of fat has a significant calorie content.

Avoiding These Foods:

Diabetes can speed up the process of plaque buildup and arterial hardening, both of which can increase a person's risk of cardiovascular disease and stroke. The following components of food can be detrimental to your efforts to maintain a diet that is good for your heart:

Fats that are saturated. Steer clear of high-fat dairy items and animal proteins like butter, beef, and processed meats like hot dogs, bacon, and sausage. Reduce your consumption of coconut and palm kernel oil as well.

Trans fats: Steer clear of processed foods, baked products, shortening, and stick kinds of margarine; these contain unhealthy trans fats.

Cholesterol: Egg yolks, liver, and other organ meats are some of the foods that are rich in cholesterol. Other sources of cholesterol include high-fat dairy products and high-fat animal proteins. Cholesterol intake should not exceed 200 milligrams (mg) per day at any point.

Sodium: Aim for a daily intake of fewer than 2,300 mg of salt. If you already have high blood pressure, your doctor may advise you to go for even lower numbers.

Putting everything into perspective: Putting together a plan. In order to assist you in maintaining a blood glucose level that is within the usual range, the diabetic diet that you construct may take one of several possible ways. You may discover, with the assistance of a dietician, that one or a combination of the following approaches is most beneficial for you:

The plate method.

A straightforward approach to meal planning is provided by the American Diabetes Association. In its most basic form, it encourages eating a greater quantity of veggies. When making your dish, make sure you follow these steps:

Vegetables that do not contain starch, such as spinach, carrots, and tomatoes, should take up half of your plate. Put some kind of protein in the bottom quarter of your plate. Some good options include chicken, pork, or tuna. Put something that has whole grains, like brown rice, or a starchy vegetable, like green peas, in the remaining one-fourth of the bowl.

Incorporate "healthy" fats into your diet in moderation, such as avocados and nuts include a portion of fruit or dairy, as well as a drink of water, unsweetened tea or coffee, and a serving of either.

Counting carbohydrates.

The largest effect on your blood glucose level is exerted by carbs because of their ability to be broken down into glucose. You might need to learn how to calculate the number of carbohydrates you eat so that you can modify the amount of insulin you take based on the results. This will help you keep better control of your blood sugar. It is essential to carefully monitor the number of carbs included in every single meal and snack.

You can learn how to accurately measure meal quantities and become an informed reader of food labels by working with a dietitian.

Additionally, he or she can instruct you on the importance of paying close attention to the portion size as well as the carbohydrate content of the food.

If you have diabetes and take insulin, a registered dietitian can show you how to count the number of carbohydrates in each meal and snack so that you can modify your insulin dosage appropriately.

Choose your foods. For the purpose of assisting you in the preparation of meals and snacks, a dietician may suggest that you choose particular foods. You have the option of selecting various foods from a list that features many categories, including carbs, proteins, and lipids. An "option" refers to a single portion available within a certain category. One serving of one food choice is equivalent to one serving of every other food in the same category in terms of the total quantity of carbohydrates, protein, and fat it contains, as well as the effect it has on your blood glucose levels. On the list of starches, fruits, and dairy products, for instance, there are several options that range from 12 to 15 grams of carbohydrates.

Glycemic index. People who have diabetes may choose their foods, particularly their sources of carbs, based on the glycemic index.

Using this strategy, you can rank foods that contain carbohydrates according to how they affect the amount of glucose in your blood. Have a discussion with your dietician to determine whether or not this approach could be beneficial to you.

A sample menu

When arranging your meal schedule, it is important to take into consideration both your size and how active you are. The menu that follows is designed for someone who needs 1,200 to 1,600 calories each day.

Breakfast. One medium slice of whole-wheat bread spread with two tablespoons of jelly, one-half cup of shredded wheat cereal mixed with one cup of 1 per cent low-fat milk, one piece of fruit, and a cup of coffee.

Lunch. A sandwich made with roast beef, lettuce, low-fat American cheese, tomato, and mayonnaise, served on wheat bread, accompanied by a medium apple and a glass of water.

Dinner. Smoked salmon, one and a half teaspoons of vegetable oil, a medium white dinner bun, one and a half cups each of carrots and green beans, a small baked potato, milk, and unsweetened iced tea, snack. 2 and a half cups of popcorn mixed with 1 and a half teaspoons of margarine.

What are the outcomes of following a diet for diabetes? Adhering to your healthy eating plan is the most effective strategy to maintain a healthy blood glucose level and reduce the risk of developing diabetes-related problems. And if you want to reduce weight, you can modify it to meet your particular needs and objectives.

A diabetes diet can provide you with a number of benefits in addition to helping you better manage your diabetes. Following a diabetes diet, which often calls for large amounts of fruits, vegetables, and fiber to be consumed, can help lower a person's chance of developing cardiovascular disease as well as several forms of cancer. In addition, consuming dairy products that are low in fat will help lower the likelihood that you will develop low bone mass in the future.

Chapter 3
The Personal Fat Threshold (PFT)

According to the 'personal fat threshold' idea, every person has a point at which they are unable to continue storing subcutaneous fat in their adipose tissue. This point varies from person to person (the fat under the skin). At this stage, fat storage in the liver and pancreas will grow, which will be followed by the development of type 2 diabetes or a worsening of the condition.

Just so there is no confusion, having a higher body mass index does not automatically result in diabetes. Instead, it's because your body fat percentage is too high in comparison to your Personal Fat Threshold. Because of their genetics and a variety of other factors that we do not yet fully understand, each individual has a unique limit to the amount of energy that they are able to comfortably store in their adipose tissue before it becomes full and causes diabetes. If this limit is exceeded, the individual will develop the condition.

The Complete Diabetes Code

Diabetes type 2 is a complicated condition, and there are a lot of different views regarding how it develops. One of these hypotheses is called the personal fat threshold hypothesis, and it proposes the following:
1. Every individual has a limit on how much fat they are able to store within the fat cells that are located beneath the skin, which is also referred to as subcutaneous fat.
2. When this threshold is reached, the body is forced to find another location in which to store the excess fat; consequently, it begins to accumulate in and around our internal organs, such as the liver and the pancreas. 3. This type of fat is known as visceral fat.
3. When this fat accumulates over time, it can have a detrimental effect on the liver's and the pancreas' ability to control the levels of glucose in the blood. The accumulation of excess visceral fat, in combination with an increase in insulin resistance, is a primary contributor to the development of type 2 diabetes and high blood sugar levels.
This theory helps explain why people of normal weight can develop type 2 diabetes as well as those who are overweight or obese.

When we go above our specific fat threshold, our bodies are no longer able to adequately handle carbohydrates and fat, which can lead to type 2 diabetes. This happens when we consume more fat than is healthy for us.

What is your own unique limit for fat intake?

At this time, there is no reliable method for determining the amount of fat that is acceptable for an individual. Additionally, there is no number that can be used as guidance for the diagnosis of this condition at this time. On the other hand, if we take a more pragmatic approach, we can define your individual fat threshold as the point at which your body begins to accumulate more fat in and around your internal organs. This is the tipping point. There are three ways that we can measure this; however, none of them is perfect:

1) Waist circumference.

This provides an estimate of the amount of fat that is stored in and around your internal organs (known as visceral fat). If it is too high, you may have already beyond the personal fat threshold for your body. In boys, "high risk" refers to a height that is greater than 94 centimeters (37 inches). Above 80 centimeters is considered tall for women (31.5in).

One thing to keep in mind is that some people will have broad waists because they undertake strength training and have a lot of muscle; nevertheless, this does not imply the same risk as having a high waist circumference owing to excess fat in the body.

2) The ratio of the waist to the hips is comparable to the circumference of the waist. This provides an indication of the amount of visceral fat you have. To determine it, take the size of your waist and divide it by the circumference of your hips. Males are deemed to be healthy and at a low risk when their ratio is 0.95 or lower. For females, the value is 0.80 or below. If you have a level that is higher than these scores, you put yourself at an increased risk of acquiring a chronic disease such as type 2 diabetes. Again, individuals who have large muscle mass levels are the exception to this rule.

3) Liver fat; unfortunately, you won't be able to simply stroll into your primary care physician's office and have the fat in your liver measured.

A scan at a medical facility or a research establishment would be required for this. However, your primary care physician will probably perform routine liver function tests, often known as LFTs, which are measurements taken from your blood.

Even while these tests won't be able to provide you with an accurate measurement of the amount of fat in your liver, they can indicate whether you might have excessive liver fat. This is because the function of your liver will become more aberrant as the amount of fat in your liver grows.

The question now is, What is the Answer?

Insulin resistance, type 2 diabetes, and metabolic syndrome are not, in and of themselves, just the outcome of consuming an excessive amount of carbohydrates in one's diet.

Instead, it's a bit more sophisticated than that, but it's still simple, and there are a few more things that need to be factored into the reason as well as the plan of action.

But if insulin and carbohydrates are not to blame for our obesity and diabetes, what can we do to combat these conditions? Is it as simple as consuming fewer calories and engaging in greater physical activity?

You might say that, but it's not quite right.

The solution to the entire conundrum may be summed up in one word: decreasing your **Personal Fat Threshold (PFT).**

How to Lose Enough Weight to Drop Below Your Individual Fat Limit

Exercising, not eating for a certain period of time (fasting), eating a nutrient-dense diet, and increasing the percentage of your diet that consists of protein.

Exercise: The hypothesis that weight loss is 80% food and 20% exercise seems to have some value.

Exercise is an adjunct that we may use to enhance insulin sensitivity and burn off fat and sugar without using insulin. While a diet rich in nutrients is the foundation for good metabolic health, exercise is an additional tool that we can employ.

The most effective forms of exercise are resistance training, activity at a lower intensity (zone 2), and bursts of activity at a higher intensity.

Fasting: A period of time spent without eating is another effective method for lowering insulin levels.

When all of the glycogen stored in your liver and muscles is used up, your body reduces the amount of insulin it produces and shifts its focus to your adipose tissue in order to release more of the fat that has been stored in your body into the system.

When it's time to refeed after a period of fasting, some people find that they easily overdo it, which might be problematic for them. When I was frequently fasting to get rid of some of the additional weight I was carrying, I discovered that I would allow myself to eat more than I normally would have. The items I selected to consume had a significantly lower nutritional density than usual but a higher energy density than usual.

Even though I was quite disciplined and stuck to my self-imposed restrictions for days on end, I didn't find that I was able to shed very much weight throughout the course of the experiment. Instead, it appeared that I was able to make up the difference in the end.

You can avoid falling into the trap of fasting for a longer period of time by guiding when and what you eat based on your glucose levels. This will ensure that you achieve a negative energy balance over the long term without pushing yourself so hard that you rebound and make poorer food choices that will undo all of your hard work.

A Higher Protein Percentage (Protein%):

A higher protein intake can assist in the development of metabolically active lean muscle mass, which can lead to an increase in resting calorie expenditure.

In addition, due to the thermic impact on food, you had the potential to increase the amount of energy (calories) you were burning when converting it into usable energy. This was possible because of the thermic effect of food (ATP).

Raising your body's overall protein content does not mean you should just consume more protein in the form that is already present in your diet.

Instead, you should focus on reducing the number of carbohydrates and dietary fats you consume while simultaneously increasing the amount of protein and fiber you take in. This will enable your body to draw fuel from its existing fat reserves.

This results in an increase in the protein percentage also referred to as the percentage of total calories that come from protein. A larger percentage of protein in your diet is associated with improved satiety, which can lead to weight loss over time.

This can be accomplished by eating a greater quantity of foods that have a lower energy density, provide a high level of satiety, and make it more difficult to consume excessive amounts of food.

This will ensure that your body's fat stores are used as fuel, which will result in a decrease in insulin levels as you continue to lose weight.

This is the reason why some people who make the conversion to a whole-food, plant-based (WFPB) diet are able to lower the amount of insulin they need and even reverse their diabetes. As long as they continue to consume only whole foods, they will be unable to consume enough calories to keep their weight stable, and their insulin levels will drop.

A Diet Rich in Nutrients Is Incomparable to Any Other Alternative!

My favorite "hack" is increasing the nutritional density as much as possible because it takes into account all of the following factors:

It offers the necessary amount of protein. You may get a sufficient amount of protein in your diet by eating foods that are rich in the vitamins, minerals, and fatty acids that are needed by your body.

If we examine each macronutrient based on the number of calories it contains, we find that protein has the highest satiety index. Protein is the subject of a great deal of misunderstanding.

However, if you consume meals that include sufficient quantities of vitamins, minerals, and fatty acids that are important to your body, you will consume an adequate amount of protein.

 On the other hand, a conscious decision to avoid protein can result in dietary shortages. Increasing the nutrient density of food, zeroing in on the macronutrients that are most likely to leave you feeling full, or placing more of an emphasis on foods that are inherently more filling all lead to the same destination: a larger sense of fullness.

It is not very dense in terms of energy. A nutrient-dense diet is one that focuses on eating complete foods that are low in energy density, have minimal levels of refined carbohydrates and processed fats, and are difficult to overeat.

It undergoes very little processing. The quantification of nutrient density is a foolproof method for ensuring that the foods you are consuming contain the essential micronutrients rather than the highly appetizing flavors and colours that Frankenfoods use to make it appear as though they are healthy for you when in reality, they are not. These minimally processed meals are filling without being overly delicious, which means that eating them will naturally reduce your food consumption.

It prevents cravings.

Finding a way to receive the nutrients you need without using an excessive amount of energy or eating a diet high in nutrients appears to be the key to warding off diabetes, maintaining a healthy weight, bringing insulin and blood glucose levels down, and regulating body weight. Your ability to feel full increases when you consume more nutrient-dense foods, which in turn makes it easier to resist cravings that unnecessarily stimulate your appetite.

Chapter 4
How to Get More Out of Life by Avoiding Diabetes

If the old saying that "an ounce of prevention is worth a pound of cure" is accurate, then there is no better time than today to begin taking steps to lower your chance of developing diabetes.

Diabetes that is not well treated might result in renal failure and perhaps blindness. It raises the likelihood that you will get significant health issues such as cardiovascular disease, limb amputation, and others.

Prevent Type 2 Diabetes

Is It Possible to Avoid Developing type 2 diabetes?

Yes! Even if you are at high risk for developing type 2 diabetes, it is possible to reduce your chance of developing the condition or put off diagnosis by making changes to your lifestyle that are scientifically supported and not overly difficult to implement.

The Complete Diabetes Code

The majority of people already have prediabetes before they develop type 2 diabetes, which means that their blood sugar is higher than normal but is not yet high enough to be diagnosed as diabetes. Prediabetes is highly prevalent; 96 million adults in the United States have it, yet more than 80 per cent of those people are unaware that they have it. The good news is that it is possible to turn prediabetes into full-blown diabetes.

According to what was covered in chapter 1, there are two different kinds of diabetes:

Insulin is a hormone that is required to allow sugar (glucose) to enter your cells and produce energy. If you have type 1 diabetes, your pancreas produces very little or no insulin, which is a condition known as diabetes type 1. Diabetes type 1, which currently has no treatment, can be caused by genetics, specific viruses, as well as other reasons. It is not possible to stop it from happening, but researchers are working on a solution.

Your pancreas will still generate some insulin even if you have type 2 diabetes, but it won't be enough to keep your body running. The uplifting news is that it is, to a significant extent, avoidable.

The Complete Diabetes Code

Despite the fact that factors like heredity, age, an unhealthy diet, and a lack of physical activity may raise your risk, there are numerous things that you can do.

Making sense of prediabetes

Diabetes and its predecessor, prediabetes, can both be diagnosed based on the levels of sugar in the blood.

The condition known as prediabetes is characterized by high blood sugar levels but does not yet meet the diagnostic criteria for diabetes.

Fortunately, alterations to one's lifestyle, as well as increased awareness of the condition, can help avoid the development of diabetes.

People who have been diagnosed with prediabetes are at a greater risk of developing type 2 diabetes than those who have not had this diagnosis.

You can sidestep this diagnosis and its complications by arming yourself with accurate information and making informed decisions about your lifestyle.

What measures can I take to lower my risk of developing diabetes?

Prevention, food, hydration, and additional support are the four areas in which efforts have the potential to bear fruit.

The Following Is a List of Natural Ways To Prevent Diabetes:

1. Stop consuming sugar and refined carbohydrates immediately.

Figure out how to differentiate between empty carbs and whole carbs. In your bloodstream, sugars and simple carbohydrates (like those present in pizza crust) are converted into glucose very quickly. Glucose is the fuel that your cells use to keep going.

This increase in blood glucose causes the production of insulin, which is a hormone that is produced in your pancreas and is responsible for transporting glucose from your bloodstream to the cells of your body.

If you have prediabetes or diabetes, your body will develop resistance to insulin, and as a result, sugar will continue to circulate through your system. Because of this, your pancreas produces even more insulin, which is the first step in the vicious cycle that is diabetes. One strategy for breaking the pattern is to reduce the amount of sugar and refined carbs that you consume.

Low-glycemic foods (those with a GI of 55 or less) do not create spikes in blood sugar and, as a result, prevent cravings from occurring. High-glycemic foods, on the other hand, cause rises in blood sugar and lead to cravings.

Consume these:

Pieces of bread and crackers are made with a variety of grains, as well as rye and sourdough.

Cereals such as rolled oats, bircher muesli, and all-bran cereals are used to make porridge. Fruits such as apples, strawberries, apricots, peaches, bananas, and kiwis vegetables such as carrots, broccoli, cauliflower, celery, tomatoes, and zucchini, sweet potatoes (especially the nutrient-rich skin), corn and yams, legumes such as chickpeas, baked beans, and kidney beans whole-grain kinds of pasta such as soba noodles, vermicelli noodles, and rice noodles nutrient-rich rice such as basmati, Doongara, long

The following types of food are not assigned a GI value because they contain very few or no carbs at all:

The meat of several kinds, including beef, chicken, hog, and lamb, as well as eggs

Nuts such as almonds, cashews, pistachios, walnuts, and macadamia nuts; fish and seafood such as salmon, trout, tuna, sardines, and shrimp; fats and oils such as olive oil, rice bran oil, butter, and margarine; herbs and spices such as salt, pepper, garlic, basil, and dill;

What about legit sugar?

There are two primary sources of sugar in the diet:

Sugars that are produced by nature, such as those that can be found in milk or fruit

Sugars are added during the processing of foods (such as the syrup that is added to canned fruit or the sugar that is added to baked products, sauces, and a wide variety of other processed foods). Be sure to give labels a close read and keep an eye out for the numerous guises sugar can take. Sugar alcohols, such as sorbitol, xylitol, and mannitol, contain fewer calories than sugars but should not be consumed on a regular basis because they are not necessarily healthful.

It is not true that a product does not include any calories or carbohydrates simply because the packaging states that it does not contain any sugar. Be sure to thoroughly inspect labels for the number of calories and grams of total carbohydrates.

Did you know?

On a nutrition label, the principal ingredients are those that appear first in the list of ingredients.

Sugar should not be labelled as the primary ingredient in any of the products that you choose to purchase. You should look for essential ingredients like whole oat flour and whole wheat flour, for example.

2. Be Portion-Conscious

Be Aware of Your Portions Individuals who are at a greater risk of getting diabetes are more likely to have raised blood sugar and insulin levels if they consume an excessive amount of food when they are eating.

The good news is that a number of studies have shown that reducing the total number of servings one consumes on a daily basis will either halt or slow down the course of diabetes.

The following is a list of straightforward approaches to reducing the size of one's portions:

Use visual references. Visualizing a serving of food in comparison to an external object, such as a tennis ball or a deck of cards, might help you gain a better idea of how much food is required to maintain good health. Eat your food carefully and pay attention to the point at which you begin to feel as though you have had enough to eat.

While you are eating, make sure to give yourself a brief rest every so often. Take your time to savor the aroma, the texture, and the flavors while you enjoy the dish!

Instead of considering these foods as the main attraction, keep in mind their potential as sauces because they are high in sugar and carbohydrates.

Consume a significant amount of water in the time leading up to each meal.

In establishments where you have no say over the portion sizes, you should always ask for a doggie bag so that you can take some of the food you ordered home with you.

When you go out to dinner with a group of people, make sure that the company you keep and the conversation you have are the highlights of the evening rather than the meal itself.

3. Eat More Fiber

The best sources of fiber come from plant-based foods. Products originating from animals do not contain the same levels of dietary fiber as those generated from plants. Adults should aim to consume anywhere between 25 and 30 grams of fiber on a daily basis.

Studies have shown that individuals who are at an increased risk of developing diabetes can benefit from lower levels of blood sugar and insulin if they consume a diet that is high in fiber. This is because fiber helps to slow the digestive process, which slows the body's production of sugar and insulin.

Dietary fiber, in addition to having positive effects on the health of the digestive tract, also has an influence on the maintenance of healthy body weight. In what ways could one possibly dislike it?

The following is a list of foods that are examples those that are rich in dietary fiber:

Beans and other types of legumes, including chickpeas, white beans, black beans, kidney beans, pinto beans, and pinto beans; lentils, and white beans. Fruits and vegetables, particularly those with edible skin (like apples) and edible seeds (like berries), should be washed whenever possible; however, you should not peel produce that has edible skin if it is still in its natural state. Examples of fruits and vegetables with edible skin and edible seeds include apples and berries.

Whole grains, such as whole-wheat pasta and whole-grain cereals, especially those having 3 grams of dietary fiber or more per serving, such as peanuts, walnuts, and almonds, are a good source of fiber. Whole grains also contain protein (but watch your portion sizes because they are calorie-rich).

Increasing the percentage of your diet that consists of raw foods can assist you in taking in a higher total fiber intake. Because the processes of cooking that soften food also reduce the amount of fiber that the food contains, you should savor the natural crunch that fruits and vegetables retain in their raw state.

4. Eat Less Food That Has Been Processed

Join in on the current trend of utilizing only a single component. It's likely that the prefabricated meals you eat, the kind that comes out of a box and includes twenty different components you can't even pronounce, are increasing your chance of acquiring heart disease, obesity, and diabetes.

Why? Since processed meals have been altered from their natural state, there is a theory that suggests they may not offer the same positive effects on one's health as whole foods.

Because of the addition of preservatives, the shelf life of processed foods can be extended; however, this does not guarantee that the item is still fresh or that it has any nutritional value.

It's likely that the problems that preservatives cause to human health won't be discovered for many years after their widespread usage has begun, especially if the preservatives in question have been kept secret. By adding sugars and fats at the end of the manufacturing process, the company tries to bring back some of the flavors that were lost during the process.

Consider making any of these adjustments to your diet in order to increase the number of whole foods you consume:

Raw fruits in their natural state, as opposed to canned or bottled processed fruit products, are preferable.

It is recommended that you use plain yoghurt as an alternative to fruit-flavoured yoghurt and then top it with sliced fruit. Homemade soups, as opposed to those made from dried components or canned products.

Guacamole is made from mashed avocados, onions, and tomatoes, rather than the pre-packaged variety bowls of taco, poke, or noodles where the toppings can be customized by the customer, as opposed to pre-packaged "make-at-home" versions of the same items guacamole made from mashed avocados, onions, and tomatoes, rather than the pre-packaged variety.

5. Make Sure You Eat a Lot of Whole Grains

Even though the white, airy Wonder Bread that was all the rage in 1921 is still on the market, that does not mean that we ought to eat it. The kinds of toast that are now available, prepared with various nutritious grains that we use for avocado toast, are substantially more worthy of our praise.

The following is a list of some of the ways in which you can improve your consumption of whole grains throughout the day:

For breakfast, you may have quinoa with a banana and almond milk, whole-grain toast with avocado or nut butter, steel-cut oats with a banana and almond milk, or whole-grain toast with a banana and almond milk. The only thing that can restrict the possible permutations is your own inventive capacity.

Bread made with whole grains is not only high in nutrients but also makes you feel extra full, so you should include it in your **noon meal.** Because they can be easily packed up and consumed in a variety of different ways, spaghetti salads that are made with whole-wheat pasta are an easy and practical option to bring to work.

Brown rice is a far healthier option than its white cousin when used as a foundation for stir-fries or as a side dish for **dinner**. Brown rice can be found in most grocery stores.

6. Step Right on Board the Ketogenic Express!

If the idea of consuming food in the same way as cavemen did appeals to you, there is a possibility that doing so will assist you in warding off the onset of diabetes.

If you follow a keto diet that is high in protein and low in carbohydrates, you will be able to improve your insulin levels and reduce the amount of fat stored in your abdominal region. You will also be given additional support in the shape of pre-prepared eating routines, things with labels, and sources of the media.

7. Stick to Water

The link between consuming beverages that are high in sugar and the development of diabetes has been unmistakably proved by scientific studies. In addition to raising the risk of developing cardiovascular disease, obesity, and a wide variety of other health conditions, they are one of the most prevalent dietary factors that can lead to the development of diabetes.

If you want to reduce your risk of acquiring diabetes in the future, you need to increase the proportion of water in your diet to other liquids if you want to keep your fluid intake at a healthy level.

Here are some tips:

Fruit can be sliced and added to water to add taste and make it more refreshing. Lemon is by far the most common citrus fruit utilized in the creation of alcoholic beverages; nonetheless, lime, orange, watermelon, berries, and even cucumber are other wonderful alternatives.

Consider making use of a pitcher that comes equipped with an infuser: You may make sparkling water at home with the help of a carbonation machine if you prefer drinking water that has bubbles and you want to save money. Place a pitcher filled with ice water inside the fridge so that it is always accessible to use.

Make your own flavored ice cubes; by placing herbs like chopped mint or basil, or even fruit that has been minced, into ice cube trays with water. Once frozen, the ice cubes may be used to give glasses of water a distinct flavor and visual appeal. You can also cut citrus fruits into slices, place them on a cookie sheet to freeze, and then store the frozen slices in a plastic bag in the freezer for use whenever you want a refreshing drink with a bit of a kick. Another option is to cut citrus fruits into wedges, place them on a cookie sheet to freeze, and then use the wedges to make a refreshing drink.

Make an investment in a water bottle that can be utilized in a number of different ways: It is important to keep in mind that sometimes what feels like hunger is really just thirst to try to pass itself off as hungry. Remembering this is especially crucial after engaging in vigorous physical activity or while travelling to an area with a high altitude. First, have something to drink, and only then should you see if there's a place for a snack.

8. Consume More Coffee and Tea: If it comes as a relief to you to realize that coffee and tea continue to play vital roles in the arsenal against diabetes, then this piece of information will come as welcome news to you.

According to the findings of a number of studies, making it a routine to consume coffee or tea on a daily basis can have a number of beneficial benefits on one's health, one of which is making it simpler to maintain control of diabetes.

Try drinking black coffee or tea with a splash of oat or almond milk instead of opting for lattes, which are known to contain a significant number of calories. If you're looking for something with a bit more pizzazz, try your hand at one of these recipes:

A matcha latte in a steaming mug Coffee flavoured with orange and cinnamon

9. Make it a Priority to Take Part in Regular Workouts That Will Make You Sweat

Exercise on a consistent basis has been shown to slow or stop the course of diabetes. Find a way to spend your time that is enjoyable to you and fits within the limits of the amount of time you have available. The most important objective is to start moving around as soon as possible and progressively extend the amount of time you spend doing so. It only takes a few minutes per day to develop a new routine.

Already a regular? You can boost the beneficial effects of your workout on your body by increasing either the intensity or the length of your workout. Aim to keep your workouts interesting by combining activities such as walking or running with strength training, swimming, or attending a class once a week. Your physician will be able to guide you in selecting the sort of exercise and the level of intensity that will be most beneficial to you.

Try using a workout app that provides you with quick access to encouragement and support from other people.

10. Strive to Achieve and Sustain a Healthy Weight (or decrease weight if your physician advises you to do so) (or lose weight if your doctor recommends it)

There are several different approaches to controlling one's weight that has been shown to be successful.

If you want to reduce a significant amount of weight or have other dietary requirements, it is highly recommended that you consult with either your primary care physician or a qualified dietitian.

Steer clear of fad diets; meal plans that consist of a single food (so long, "cottage cheese diet"), and other weight loss strategies that promise outcomes that are too good to be true (ahem, the "sleep diet").

Instead, make it a goal to eat a variety of whole, unprocessed foods that are cooked without the addition of any extra sweets or carbohydrates.

Take into consideration the following eating regimens, which are more suited to your lifestyle:

Mediterranean diet. A way of eating is based on the decreased incidence of heart disease that is seen in persons who live in Mediterranean countries.

Low-carb diet. A diet that reduces the number of carbohydrates consumed and places more emphasis on the consumption of healthy fats. Diets such as the ketogenic diet and its more well-known predecessor, the Atkins diet, are both good examples.

Paleo diet. A diet that consists primarily of foods like fish, lean meats, fruits, vegetables, nuts, and seeds (consider the kinds of foods that our predecessors who lived in caves might have obtained by hunting and gathering) (think of foods our cave-dwelling ancestors would have obtained by hunting and gathering). Milk products, legumes, and grains are restricted or eliminated from the diet.

Pescatarian diet. If you want to increase your consumption of omega-3 fatty acids, zinc, calcium, and protein—all nutrients that have been related to preventing diabetes—incorporate fish and shellfish into your vegetarian diet (all nutrients linked to diabetes prevention).

A buildup of fat around the abdominal organs, also known as visceral fat, is associated with a number of significant health risks, including insulin resistance. Despite the fact that there is no scientifically proven method to lose weight from only one part of your body, you should be aware of this risk.

If you have a lower waistline, you may be able to avoid some health problems, such as diabetes.

11. Get More Exercise

There is a clear correlation between leading a sedentary lifestyle and developing diabetes, according to large-scale observational research.

Find ways to make activities that you normally perform while sitting or standing still into ones that need you to move around.

Here are some suggestions that will help you begin moving:

Listen to music that makes you want to dance while you clean the house (a broom or mop makes a terrific dance partner!).

Walk while talking to members of your family and close friends on the phone.

While you're waiting on hold, strike a stance (yoga pose) (you may need to use a speakerphone) (speakerphone may be necessary).

You should remind yourself to get up and move about every 90 minutes by setting the alarm on either your computer or your phone.

Use a standing desk.

Instead of taking the elevator, you should use the steps.

Park your vehicle further away from the entrances of stores and your place of business.

Altering your behavior may at first seem challenging, but after some time has passed, you will find that it has become natural to you.

12. Stop Smoking

Numerous studies have found a connection between active and passive smoking and the onset and progression of diabetes in both males and females.

There are a lot of good reasons to give up smoking, and there are a lot of different ways to seek support.

Get more information by talking to your local doctor or attending meetings of groups that help people quit smoking.

13. Get Your Vitamin D

Vitamin D is a superhero when it comes to blood sugar. Having low levels of vitamin D has been linked in a number of studies to an increased risk of developing both kinds of diabetes.

Breaking news: Your smartphone, in contrast to the sun, does not release the UV rays that are necessary for your body to produce vitamin D.

If you are unable to spend time outside, consider including in your diet some of the following foods that are rich in vitamin D: Swordfish, salmon, or tuna, enriched milk, yoghurt, and cheese made with fortified milk, beef liver, and egg yolks are some of the foods that are recommended. Cereals that have been fortified, particularly low-sugar, whole-grain variants

Have a discussion about taking a vitamin D supplement with your primary care physician. They are available in both tablet and capsule form. Ongoing studies investigate whether vitamin D can help prevent diabetes and lessen its symptoms in those who already have the disease.

14. Go on Nature

It is believed that certain naturally occurring chemicals can lower your risk of developing diabetes.

Turmeric, a spice that is commonly used in Indian cuisine, contains a compound called curcumin as its primary active component. Turmeric is known to have characteristics that reduce inflammation in the body, in addition to imparting an amazing flavor to the cuisine. Berberine is a plant extract that is consumed orally and has the potential to assist in the regulation of how the body utilizes sugar.

Always consult your primary care physician before beginning a new dietary supplement. It's possible that the herbal supplements you take could interact negatively with the prescriptions you're already on.

15. Mind Your Mental Health and Take Care of It

According to the findings of the study, being depressed may make one more susceptible to getting type 2 diabetes. It is just as vital to manage your mental health as it is to manage your diet and your exercise level.

16. Maintain Your Connections

Despite the fact that there is currently no treatment for diabetes, research is continuing. Make it a priority to stay current on the various therapy alternatives.

Attend a cooking class or look for online support groups that focus on healthy eating. Explore new dining establishments that provide menu items with a focus on health. In addition, make it a habit to visit your primary care physician on a regular basis so he or she can keep an eye on any risk factors or other health concerns you may have.

The Botom Line

You are the one who decides how sweet your life will be. You might not be able to manage everything that makes diabetes a danger, but you are in charge of a good deal of the risk factors, which is a really empowering position to be in.

Get into the zone, and you won't have to worry about diabetes again! Develop a strategy for healthy food, choose wisely when it comes to beverages, commit to leading an active lifestyle, and benefit from the support that we have just outlined!

Summary

Insulin is a hormone that is produced by the pancreas. It allows glucose, which comes from food, to enter the cells of the body. When there is not enough insulin or when cells cease responding to insulin, an excessive amount of blood sugar remains in the bloodstream. If you have type 1 diabetes, you will need to inject insulin into your body every day in order to stay alive. Type 2 diabetes affects adults more frequently than children and accounts for 90 per cent of all occurrences of diabetes.

Diabetes that develops during pregnancy may typically disappear after the delivery of the baby. Diabetes type 1 can develop at any point in a person's life. At any age, a person is at risk for developing type 2 diabetes. Both type 1 and type 2 may have their origins in a complex web of hereditary and environmental risk factors. It is currently uncertain what exactly causes the majority of kinds of diabetes.

Diabetes can produce difficulties and health problems that have the potential to make depressive symptoms more severe. Having a history of depression has been linked to an increased risk of acquiring type 2 diabetes.

Both diabetes and depression are treatable diseases that can benefit from lifestyle adjustments and different medications. The risk of developing type 1 diabetes can be increased by both environmental and geographical variables. Certain persons, such as those who are Black, Hispanic, American Indian, or Asian American, are at a higher risk.

Diabetes can cause nerve damage (neuropathy), which can destroy the walls of the capillaries in the blood vessels supplying nutrition to the nerves. Diabetes can cause eye damage and nerve damage to the retina, which could lead to permanent vision loss. Diabetes type 2 has been linked to an increased chance of developing dementia, including Alzheimer's disease. The vast majority of healthy babies are delivered by mothers who have gestational diabetes. The same changes in lifestyle that can help cure prediabetes and type 2 diabetes can also help avoid these conditions, according to the American Diabetes Association (ADA).

If you are overweight, decreasing as little as 7% of your body weight can significantly reduce the likelihood that you will get diabetes. A person who weighs 200 pounds (90.7 kilograms) may be able to reduce their chance of developing diabetes by dropping 14 pounds (6.4 kilograms).